Refraction and Retinoscopy: How to Pass the Refraction Certificate

JONATHAN C PARK
BSc (Hons), MB ChB (Hons), FRCOphth
Ophthalmic Specialty Training Registrar
South West Peninsula Deanery

and

DAVID H JONES
MA, BM BCh, FRCOphth
Consultant Ophthalmologist
Royal Cornwall Hospital

Illustrations supervised by
SALMAN WAQAR
BSc, MBBS, MRCS (Ed)
Ophthalmic Specialty Training Registrar
South West Peninsula Deanery

Foreword by
ANTHONY QUINN
Consultant Ophthalmologist
Head of School, Ophthalmology
NHS South West Peninsula Deanery

Radcliffe Publishing
London • New York

Radcliffe Publishing Ltd
33–41 Dallington Street
London
EC1V 0BB
United Kingdom

www.radcliffehealth.com

British Library Cataloguing in Publication Data

A catalogue record for this book is available from the British Library.

ISBN-13: 978 190891 191 9

The paper used for the text pages of this book is FSC® certified. FSC (The Forest Stewardship Council®) is an international network to promote responsible management of the world's forests.

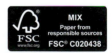

Typeset by Darkriver Design, Auckland, New Zealand
Printed and bound by Hobbs the Printers, Totton, Hants, UK

Guidance regarding common errors

Whilst revising for the Refraction Certificate, it is important to consider the feedback provided to the ophthalmic trainees group in April 2011.

The most common errors included:

- indecipherable numbers
- incorrect nomenclature (for example, not using + or – signs)
- forgetting to record visual acuity
- incorrect transposition from retinoscopy prescription
- final refraction written down incorrectly, despite correct initial workings
- inability to refract quickly under pressure (reflecting that failure is related to inexperience).

Therefore, it would be wise to practise adequately prior to the examination and ensure that your recordings are precise and correct.

3

What does refractive error mean?

Ametropia

Emmetropia

'Emmetropia' means the absence of a refractive error, so light from a distant source is perfectly focused on the retina (*see* Figure 3.1). An emmetrope will have normal distance acuity with no spectacles (uncorrected Snellen acuity of 6/6 or better) – provided, of course, there is no amblyopia, ocular pathology or cerebral visual impairment.

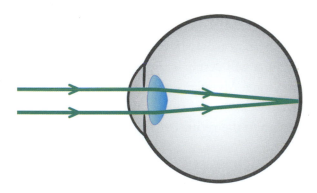

FIGURE 3.1 Emmetropia: light from a distant object forms an image on the retina

Refractive error (ametropia)

'Refractive error' (ametropia) means that an eye does not allow light from a distant source to be focused perfectly on the retina. Approximately one-third of the population has a refractive error of more than 1 dioptre, and thus may need spectacles. Myopia is just as common as hypermetropia.

The refractive power of an eye is a function of the corneal curvature (accounting for two-thirds of the power; this cannot be altered) and lens (accounting for one-third of the power; this can be altered by accommodation, provided there is no presbyopia). This is a surprise to most people, since most assume that the lens is the most powerful refractive element. The air–cornea interface is in fact the most powerful refractive element – this becomes quite obvious when you dive into water without any goggles.

> Refractive error (ametropia) occurs when the refractive power of the eye does not correlate with the axial length of the eye, so an image from a distant object does not fall on the retina.

Myopia

'Myopia' (short-sightedness) means that the refractive power of the eye is too great relative to the axial length of the eye; as a result, the image of a distant object lies in front of the retina (*see* Figure 3.2). Therefore, myopia will result if the refractive power is too high or if the eye is too long. Myopia is corrected by a minus (concave) lens, which effectively weakens the refractive power to allow the image to be shifted back on to the retina (*see* Figure 3.3).

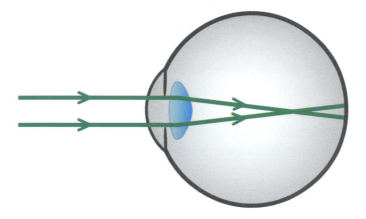

FIGURE 3.2 Myopia: light from a distant object forms an image in front of the retina

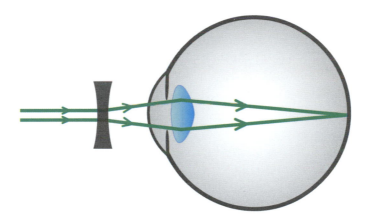

FIGURE 3.3 Myopia corrected by a minus (concave) lens that diverges rays

Hypermetropia

'Hypermetropia' (long-sightedness) means that the refractive power of the eye is too weak relative to the axial length of the eye; as a result, the image of a distant object lies behind the retina (*see* Figure 3.4). Therefore, hypermetropia will result if the refractive power is too low, or if the eye is too short. Hypermetropia is corrected by a plus (convex) lens, which effectively strengthens the refractive power to allow the image to be shifted forwards on to the retina (*see* Figure 3.5).

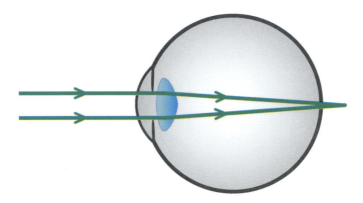

FIGURE 3.4 Hypermetropia – light from a distant object forms an image behind the retina

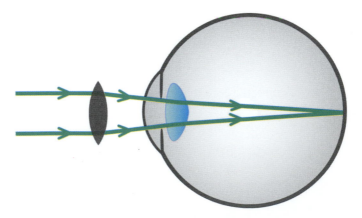

FIGURE 3.5 Hypermetropia corrected by a plus (convex) lens that converges rays

4

How to refract

Overview

There are different ways to refract a patient (i.e. to obtain a spectacle prescription to correct refractive error). We detail a system that can be practised to correctly refract a patient and obtain all the necessary information required to complete the Refraction Certificate Examination (at the time of writing).

Refracting a patient takes as long as it takes; however, the majority of cases can be refracted within 15 to 20 minutes. Practise is required and the system following provides a framework for this, which you can modify if necessary, according to the advice you are provided with whilst training. You will need to refract 70 to 100 patients before feeling comfortable with most situations and hence before you can pass the Refraction Certificate Examination.

Remember that the certificate OSCE consists of multiple stations, so different parts of the refractive process may be examined in various different orders. However, as already discussed, we have arranged these parts in an order that makes clinical sense. For example, the stations listed under 'Refraction of an adult' are those typically used to refract an adult in sequence from start to finish, which, as noted, typically takes 15 to 20 minutes.

Note that 'objective refraction' implies obtaining a refractive prescription that does not require any response from the patient – this is obtained by retinoscopy; for children or adults with learning disability, this may be the sole basis for a spectacle prescription.

'Subjective refraction' relates to fine-tuning the prescription obtained from retinoscopy by asking the patient a number of clear, closed questions whilst avoiding fatigue. This is where the art of refraction becomes evident!

The refractive process

The following is a useful template of the refractive process undertaken with an adult, which should take approximately 20 minutes. Once experienced, it can take considerably less time, as the examination can be tailored to fit the patient; however, for the purpose of the Refraction Certificate Examination, all components must be well rehearsed.

History (2 minutes).

IPD/Trial frame/Back vertex distance (BVD) (1 minute).

Visual acuity (2 minutes).

Objective refraction – retinoscopy (5–10 minutes).
- Typically without cycloplegia in an adult.

Subjective refraction (5–10 minutes).
- Sphere.
- Cyl axis.
- Cyl power and sphere compensation.
- Duochrome.
- Binocular balance.
- MR and PCT.
- Near vision.

Recording results (1 minute).

History

This should be brief – about 2 minutes. Introduce yourself then ask the patient for their name and age. Clinically, it is useful to ask the following:

'Do you wear spectacles or contact lenses?'
'Are your spectacles single vision, bifocal or varifocal?'
- If bifocal or varifocal, presbyopia is relevant, so you will need a near add.

'At what age did you start wearing spectacles?'
- The younger the age, often the greater the refractive error and higher the chance of amblyopia.

'When do you wear your spectacles – when looking into the distance (such as when driving/watching television) or at things close by (e.g. when reading)?'
- A mild myope may only wear them for distance.
- An emmetrope or mild hypermetrope who is older than 35 years (presbyopia may start to manifest from this point) may only wear them for reading.

'Are you a driver?'
- If so, their best corrected binocular visual acuity should be better than 6/12, which approximates the Driver and Vehicle Licensing Agency's legal requirement of being able to read a number plate with both eyes open at a distance of 20 metres away.

'What is your occupation/hobby?'
- Computer work may require a specific intermediate correction (a weaker near add to the distance prescription than that required for reading).

'Do you do anything that requires you to see objects closer than at normal reading distance, such as sewing/model making?'
- A stronger near add may be needed for such closer work.

'Have you had any eye problems in the past?'
- Has there been any surgery, laser, trauma or drops?
- Have there been any problems with a lazy eye/use of patch as a child?
  - Amblyopia or previous eye disease may limit best corrected visual acuity, so do not panic if 6/6 is not obtained in these cases.

'Do you have any double vision – where you see two images?'
- Patients may report blurred vision as double vision – always establish if two separate images are seen (true diplopia) and whether this is binocular (suggesting a squint without suppression) or monocular (suggesting unilateral ocular pathology such as a cataract or corneal scar).
- For binocular diplopia, it is important to assess the squint angle with the cover test and MR, and the patient may require prisms for their symptoms.

Inter-pupillary distance, trial frame and back vertex distance

It should only take a minute or two to measure the inter-pupillary distance (IPD), fit the trial frame and measure the back vertex distance (BVD).

Inter-pupillary distance

Ask the patient to look at a distant target and measure the distance from the right nasal limbus to their left temporal limbus using a rule (which you should bring yourself to the exam). The IPD typically lies between 55 and 75 mm.

Inter-pupillary distance near

Check you are at the same height as the patient. Face the patient and ask them to look at your open eye (close your right eye; with your left eye, measure from their right nasal limbus) then ask them to look at your other eye (now close your left eye, open your right eye and measure to their left temporal limbus). Typically, the IPD for near is 2 to 4 mm less than for distance due to the convergence that occurs with near stimulation.

Fit trial frame

Set your trial frame IPD to the distance IPD value you have just measured. Make the side arms as long as possible then place on the frame on the patient's face, checking that the side arms hook around the ears and tighten the side arms until stable and comfortable. Check that the pupil is easily seen – if it is obscured in the horizontal plane, you will need to re-check your IPD; if it is obscured in the vertical plane, you will need to adjust the nasal rest (if the pupil is too high, lower the central frame bracket to elevate the trial frame, *see* Figure 4.1).

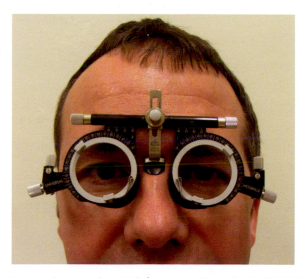

FIGURE 4.1 Correct fitting of a trial frame with each pupil in the centre of each aperture, both horizontally and vertically.

Back vertex distance

Place a lens (of any value) in the trial frame. Ask the patient to fixate on a distant target, and use a rule to measure from the patient's cornea to the back of the lens (the surface of the lens nearest the cornea). A normal BVD is 10 to 12 mm.

The power of a lens system depends upon the distance of the lens from the cornea. This concept is known as 'lens effectivity' and explains why a myope's contact lens prescription will be numerically weaker than their spectacle prescription. It also explains why patients with powerful prescriptions get a blurred view when their spectacles slip down their nose.

Therefore, the BVD is important when a frame is to be constructed, since the function of the lens system depends not only on the lens power but also on the lens position relative to the cornea. Practically, this is relevant for prescriptions of more than 4 dioptres, but it is good practice to always record the BVD. Formulae exist to allow correction of any given prescription as well as BVD to a different prescription and BVD that will have an equivalent effect.

Visual acuity

'Acuity' is a measure of the resolving power of the eye – the ability to discriminate between two points. Distance charts that you should be comfortable with include the Snellen and the LogMAR. Near vision charts that you should be comfortable with include the N-series.

In any clinical setting, it is important to check the distance visual acuity for each eye (unaided, aided and pinhole) and the near acuity for each eye (unaided and aided). If aided, it is useful to state if this is with spectacles or contact lenses. The eye not being tested should be correctly occluded.

For the purpose of the exam, the patient's spectacles will not be available, so the following will need to be established for each eye:
- distance acuity unaided (Snellen or LogMAR)

- distance acuity with pinhole
- near acuity unaided (N-series; remember to use a bright lamp).

Pinholes only allow axial rays through to the eye, hence reduce the effect of refractive error. Remember that the pinhole vision gives a good idea of potential vision for that eye once the refractive error has been corrected. Ideally, your target end-refraction visual acuity should be at least as good as the pinhole acuity.

Remember that eyes with reduced pinhole vision or reduced vision despite adequate refractive correction have acuity that is limited by amblyopia, ocular pathology or cerebral visual impairment. Pinhole acuity tends to partially improve with corneal or lens pathology but will not improve with amblyopia, retinal, nerve or cerebral pathology (pinhole acuity can be worse than unaided acuity in patients with macular pathology, since it precludes eccentric fixation).

Always consider – why is the vision poor?

Refractive error:
. . . improves with pinhole.

Amblyopia:
. . . no improvement with pinhole.

Ocular pathology:
. . . if of retina or nerve origin, will not improve with pinhole
. . . if of cornea or lens origin, may improve with pinhole.

Cerebral visual impairment:
. . . no improvement with pinhole.

Note, of course, a mixture of these reasons commonly coexist.

Refraction estimation

Checking the visual acuity will give you an idea of the refractive error:

- 1 dioptre of spherical error gives 6/12
- 2 dioptres of spherical error give 6/24 to 6/36
- 3 dioptres of spherical error give 6/60.

However, note that this guide is for spherical error and ignores that the patient may have astigmatism. The impairment in acuity is about half that for cylindrical errors relative to spherical errors. Therefore, a patient with 0.00/+2.00 @ 080 would be approximately 6/12 unaided.

This guide should only be used as an approximation, since patients will have a mixture of spherical and cylindrical error.

This refraction estimation alone does not, however, suggest whether the patient is myopic or hypermetropic. For example, if they are 6/24 unaided, their refraction could be –1.75 or +1.75 spherical dioptres. To estimate if the patient is myopic or hypermetropic, compare their unaided distance acuity with their unaided near acuity. This concept is more useful if the patient is presbyopic, since otherwise the effect of accommodation confounds the estimation. If a patient has poor distance vision but good near vision, you know they are myopic. For example, if a presbyope has an unaided Snellen distance acuity of 6/60, yet is N5 at reading distance (on the near vision N-series reading chart), their refraction is probably around –2.00 to –3.00 spherical dioptres.

If they have poor distance vision and poor near vision, you know they are hypermetropic (or they have amblyopia, or ocular pathology or cerebral visual impairment – this should be clear from your history).

Visual acuity testing of a child

Although children can be unpredictable, which adds stress to an examination setting since it is something you cannot control, there are a number of useful ways of handling this that come with experience in assessing the visual behaviour of children.

It is important to spend time with orthoptic staff, since this is the best way to learn to be comfortable with the following:

- patching as a means of occlusion (note that objection to occlusion implies poor acuity in the other eye)
- assessing if a child's vision is central (i.e. no squint), steady (i.e. conjugate movements with no nystagmus) and maintained through the duration of a blink (i.e. there is sufficient acuity to fixate on and follow an object of interest, demonstrating that it is seen)
- preselected tests, such as Cardiff Cards, Kay Pictures, single optotype or crowded charts, used to assess binocular and monocular distance acuity.

Retinoscopy (objective refraction)

Retinoscopy basics

The aim of retinoscopy is to obtain an objective refraction – that is, an estimation of the patient's spectacle prescription using a process that does not require any decisions to be made by the patient.

Retinoscopy also gives a good benchmark from which the prescription can be fine-tuned using subjective techniques (using subjective rather than objective refraction from the beginning takes considerably longer).

Retinoscopy is an invaluable process for children or adults with learning disability, as these patients will not be able to answer the questions required for subjective refraction. For these patients, your spectacle prescription will be based on your retinoscopy alone.

A retinoscope produces a light, which, with the cuff fully down, is linear (the scope slit). For more information on the retinoscope, *see* Appendix 2. Quite simply, the scope slit light is passed across the patient's pupil and a light within the pupil (the reflex) is observed. By noting the quality of this reflex, various lenses are then placed in the trial frame to neutralise the reflex. As neutralisation is approached, the reflex will become faster and brighter. A dull, slow reflex implies neutralisation is not close. At neutralisation, the reflex is a glowing bright pupil; at this point, the lenses in the trial frame provide the objective spectacle prescription (once corrected for working distance).

The scope slit is held at a certain angle (say, vertically) then swept across the pupil in a direction perpendicular to the orientation of the scope slit (in this case, horizontally). As the scope slit passes across the pupil, the reflex can be noted to have certain characteristics: (a) direction, (b) orientation, and (c) brightness and speed.

Characteristics of retinoscope reflex

Direction:
- *with* or *against* or neutralised.

Orientation:
- vertical, horizontal or oblique
- scissor reflex.

Brightness and speed:
- bright and fast
- dull and slow.

Direction of reflex

A 'with' reflex is seen if, as your slit passes across the pupil, a light within the pupil (the reflex) moves in the same direction (*see* Figure 4.2). A *plus lens must be added* to the trial frame to approach neutralisation.

An 'against' reflex is seen if, as your slit passes across the pupil, a light within the pupil (the reflex) moves in the opposite direction (*see* Figure 4.3). A *minus lens must be added* to the trial frame to approach neutralisation.

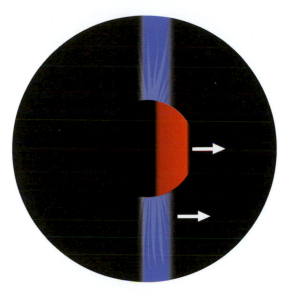

FIGURE 4.2 A 'with' reflex. The scope slit is orientated vertically and swept horizontally across the pupil to give a *with* reflex

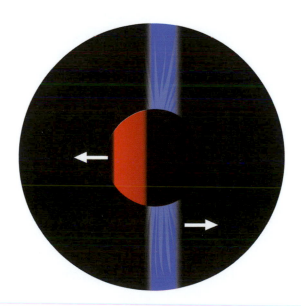

FIGURE 4.3 An 'against' reflex. The scope slit is orientated vertically and swept horizontally across the pupil to give an *against* reflex

> To neutralise:
>
> *with* reflex . . . add plus lens
> *against* reflex . . . add minus lens.

Therefore, to approach neutralisation, either a plus (if *with* reflex) or minus (if *against* reflex) must be added to the trial frame. If the reflex is already quite fast and bright, only 0.25 or 0.50 may be sufficient to reach neutralisation. To confirm neutralisation, you can lean backwards, further away from the patient (reflex becomes *against*) or lean forwards closer to the patient (reflex becomes *with*). This is because the closer you are, the more minus must be added to correct for the working distance (*see* 'Correction for working distance', p. 34). Alternatively, to ensure the end point has been reached, add a +0.25 lens, which should give an *against* reflex. Such reversal of the reflex is important to achieve, since it highlights that the true end point of neutralisation has been established.

Note that the lenses added to approach neutralisation are either spherical or cylindrical. If a sphere is added to neutralise the reflex, it will also alter the subsequent lenses required in the perpendicular axis to obtain neutralisation. If a cylindrical lens is added (with the axis orientated the same way as the scope slit, so the power of the cylindrical lens will act in the same plane as the scope sweep), neutralisation in this plane is approached and has no effect on the other principal meridian.

Orientation of reflex

> The orientation of the retinoscope's slit light should be parallel to the pupil reflex.

If there is no astigmatism, or if the astigmatism is either with the rule or against the rule, the reflex will be orientated vertically and horizontally. In these situations, ensure the slit is vertical then horizontal (rotate the slit by rotating the cuff slightly) to neutralise these meridians.

With oblique astigmatism, the principal meridians are still perpendicular but do not lie vertically and horizontally. Therefore, when a horizontal scope sweep is made with the slit orientated vertically, the orientation of the pupil reflex will be oblique and not lie vertically (it will lie between 045 and 090 or 090 and 135) – *see* Figure 4.4. Similarly, if the scope slit was orientated horizontally and a sweep made vertically, the orientation of the pupil reflex will again be oblique and not be horizontal (it will lie between 000 and 045 or 135 and 180). For oblique astigmatism, the scope slit should be rotated by turning the cuff slightly so the slit is parallel to the pupil reflex to aid subsequent neutralisation. The perpendicular meridian can then be neutralised by rotating the slit 90 degrees (e.g. if one meridian is at 110, the other will be at 020).

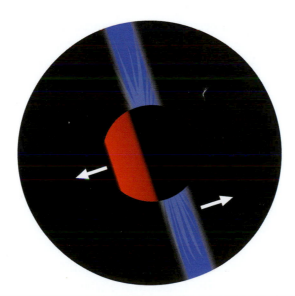

FIGURE 4.4 With oblique astigmatism, the orientation of the reflex will not be horizontal or vertical but oblique

Another type of reflex is the 'scissor reflex', which occurs with a high degree of irregular corneal astigmatism, such as keratoconus. These reflexes can be difficult or simply not possible to neutralise. Keratoconus is a corneal ectasia, characterised by progressive stromal thinning and conical distortion, associated with increasing irregular astigmatism and myopia. It is appropriate to examine the eye on the slit lamp for other signs of keratoconus (stromal thinning/cone, Vogt's striae, Fleischer ring). Investigations include corneal topography so the degree of irregular astigmatism can be quantified and mapped. This aids the consideration of the various available treatment options for keratoconus, including contact lenses, scleral contact lenses or surgical intervention (riboflavin with ultraviolet A/collagen cross-linking, intra-stromal implants, deep lamellar or penetrating keratoplasty).

Brightness and speed of reflex

As mentioned, the brighter and faster the reflex, the closer to neutralisation. In these situations, use a small magnitude of lens power alteration (0.25 or 0.50 dioptres) since neutralisation is close.

Therefore, a dull, slow reflex is far from neutralisation and sometimes it pays to begin with a ±5 or ±10 spherical lens to start off with.

Remember, a dull reflex also occurs with medial opacity (such as with a cataract or vitreous haemorrhage). A dull reflex can also occur as a result of flat retinoscope batteries!

Correction for working distance

'Working distance' is the distance from the patient's cornea to your retinoscope.

It is necessary to alter the sphere of the lenses in the trial frame to give a corrected full prescription based upon the value of the working distance.

The retinoscope is constructed so that if retinoscopy is performed at 1 m from the patient, the lenses in the trial frame to give neutralisation are equal to the spectacle prescription. However, we do not do retinoscopy at 1 m, but rather at 66 cm (when working with trial

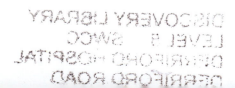

frames) or 50 cm (if you have shorter arms or when working without trial frames – for example, with children, examination under anaesthesia or a model eye). Therefore, once neutralisation is obtained, to convert to the corrected prescription, it is necessary to add a –1.50 sphere to the trial frame (to correct for a 66 cm working distance) or a –2.00 sphere (to correct for a 50 cm working distance). Note that the cyl remains unchanged.

Therefore, a –1.50 myope will neutralise without any lenses if working at 66 cm. A –2.00 myope will neutralise without any lenses if working at 50 cm.

Here are some other examples:

- neutralisation occurs with +4.25/–1.75 @ 030 at 66 cm, so the corrected refraction will be +2.75/–1.75 @ 030, since +4.25 plus –1.50 = +2.75
- neutralisation occurs with –3.75/+0.75 @ 044 at 50 cm, so the corrected refraction will be –5.75/+0.75 @ 044, since –3.75 plus –2.00 = –5.75.

> Therefore, the working distance correction factor is the reciprocal of the working distance in metres and this must be subtracted from the retinoscopy result.
>
> Whenever a result is recorded, it is vital to state whether this is uncorrected or corrected for the working distance and what that working distance is. Therefore, add a –1.50 spherical lens for a working distance of 66 cm and add a –2.00 spherical lens for a working distance of 50 cm.

The correction of working distance can be done at the end of the retinoscopy once neutralisation has been achieved, whilst working at 66 cm or 50 cm. However, it can be done at the start of retinoscopy. In this case, before using the retinoscope, you must add +1.50 (for 66 cm) or +2.00 (for 50 cm) to the trial frame (or your fingers, if working with no frame), and the resultant lens summation at neutralisation will give the corrected prescription. Whether you decide to correct for working distance at the end or the start of retinoscopy does not matter – but it must be done and your results should be clearly recorded to demonstrate at what stage a correction for working distance was made.

Static versus dynamic retinoscopy

'Static' retinoscopy means that the working distance is fixed throughout retinoscopy. This is what most practice and is what is detailed in this book.

Experienced practitioners can use the concept of working distance to their advantage by varying their working distance to obtain neutralisation (rather than changing the lenses). This is known as 'dynamic' retinoscopy.

For example, an emmetrope neutralises at 1 m, a −1.50 myope at 66 cm, a −2.00 myope at 50 cm, a −5.00 myope at 20 cm and so on. Imagine you get an against movement at 66 cm – rather than adding a minus lens (in the case of static retinoscopy), you instead lean forward to 50 cm and neutralisation occurs – the patient's refraction in that meridian is therefore −2.00.

Dynamic retinoscopy is less practical for hypermetropes, since hypermetropes neutralise with a working distance of more than 1 m.

Dynamic retinoscopy takes considerable practise but is extremely useful for refracting challenging patients (such as children) because it is so rapid.

Retinoscopy technique

Ideally, the room should be dim. The darker the room, the easier it is to note the reflex characteristics; if the room is too dark, you will struggle to find your lenses. A useful trick is to use your retinoscope light as a torch if you cannot see the lens markings easily.

Ensure that your retinoscope cuff is all the way down on the shaft of the retinoscope.

Key points for retinoscopy

- Establish a dim room.
- Fog (or occlude, if necessary) the fellow eye.
- Scope the patient's right eye with your right eye/right hand.
- Scope the patient's left eye with your left eye/left hand.
- Keep your scope as close as possible to their visual axis, without interrupting continuous distant fixation.
- Correct for working distance (add −1.50 sphere if at 66 cm; add −2.00 sphere if at 50 cm).
- Record in either positive cyl notation for both eyes or negative cyl notation for both eyes (never positive for one eye and negative for the other).

The first step is to examine the patient's right eye with the retinoscope. For non-cycloplegic refraction of patients who are not presbyopic (especially if they are myopic), it is necessary to fog (blur) the fellow left eye. This involves placing a +1.50 or +2.00 spherical lens on top of the presumed refraction (estimated from their acuity, which you have just checked), so that the acuity is poorer than that of the eye being examined with the retinoscope.

Adequate fogging can be confirmed by ensuring that the retinoscopy reflex is against or, alternatively, checking the acuity in each eye with the fog in place and ensuring the fogged eye has poorer acuity than the eye about to be objectively refracted. If the patient is 6/6 with the presumed refraction, a +1.50 or +2.00 spherical dioptre fog typically renders the eye to 6/12 to 6/24.

The reason why the fellow eye should be fogged is to reduce accommodation, which would give a false result when examining the fellow eye with the retinoscope. With cycloplegic refraction (typically in children), there is no need to fog, since the accommodative

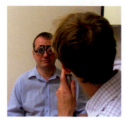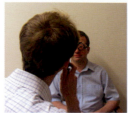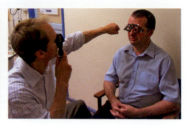

FIGURE 4.5 Use your left hand to perform retinoscopy of the patient's left eye (left photo), since incorrectly using your right hand will obstruct their view (central photo). Check working distance with arm (right photo).

component is removed by the cycloplegia. For non-cycloplegic refraction (most adults), fogging is required to reduce any accommodative drive (especially if the patient is a myope who is not yet presbyopic).

This fogging induces less accommodation than simple occlusion with a black occluder – hence, the effort made to fog rather than simply occlude.

Occlusion, rather than fogging, should be avoided, as it stimulates more accommodation. However, occlusion is required in the following situations:

- when the eye being tested is densely amblyopic (since the eye not being tested must have a poorer acuity to help avoid accommodation and a +2.00 lens will probably be insufficient to achieve this)
- if the patient markedly objects to fogging due to diplopia or asthenopia
- if you are unable to estimate acuity and provide an adequate fog lens.

Once you have adequately fogged (or, if necessary, occluded) the fellow eye, ask the patient to fixate on the white light or green target in the distance. Explain to them that it is important that they continue to look into the distance and not at your own white light. Ask them to let you know if your head obscures their view of the distant fixation target. It is vital to ensure that your head is as close as possible to their visual axis, without actually obscuring their distant fixation target – this ensures that your retinoscope light will be close to their visual axis (*see* Figure 4.5). Failure to be 'on axis' in this way can result in spurious astigmatism, thus it is important to be wary of this when refracting children who shift their position.

Use your right hand and right eye to scope their right eye. Scope first with a vertical, then a horizontal and finally a diagonal slit to locate the principal meridians. If only a dull, slow reflex is seen, try using a ±5 or even a ±10 lens. Then proceed by refracting in plus or minus cyls or spheres alone (*see* 'Working in plus/minus cyls or spheres', p. 39).

Once you have objectively refracted the right eye, correct for your working distance (add a –1.50 sphere if at 66 cm) and record your result (state 'corrected for working distance'). Then fog the right eye and use your left hand and left eye to scope their left eye. Once you have objectively refracted the left eye, again correct for working distance and record this. You should now turn the lights on, check the visual acuity and move onto subjective refraction.

Remember that if a *with* reflex is seen, then a plus lens should be added and if an *against* reflex is seen then a minus lens should be added to approach neutralisation. The brighter and faster the reflex, the closer you are to neutralisation (the entire pupil lights up when the slit enters the pupil), whereas a dull and slow reflex implies you are not close to neutralisation.

Working in plus/minus cyls or spheres

It is possible to refract with your retinoscope in three different ways:
1   using positive cyls
2   using negative cyls
3   using spheres only.

Using positive cyls

This means that your retinoscopy result will be in a plus cyl format.

Identify the orientation of the two principal meridians, which will be perpendicular to each other. The principal meridian that has an *against* reflex – or, if both reflexes are *with*, it will be the least *with* reflex (which is fastest and brightest, as it is nearest neutralisation) – is neutralised first with spheres. This will result in the other principal meridian giving a *with* reflex, which is then neutralised with positive cyls (the axis on the lens in the same orientation as the scope slit). The resultant prescription will be the lenses in the trial frame (which must then be corrected for working distance).

For example, you identify an *against* reflex with scope slit at 135 and a *with* reflex at 045. Add minus spheres until the *against* reflex at 135 is neutralised (say, –3.00 causes neutralisation). Then add plus cyls (with the axis in the same orientation as the scope slit at 045) to neutralise the *with* reflex (say, +1.50 at 045 causes neutralisation). The axis line on the cyl lens should be parallel to the scope slit and light reflex (perpendicular to its power). The lenses in the trial frame then give the retinoscopy result in plus cyl format: –3.00/+1.50 @ 045, which must then be corrected for working distance (if at 66 cm, this gives –4.50/+1.50 @ 045).

This may sound complicated, but simply consider that a patient with regular astigmatism requires a sphere with a cyl superimposed upon it to correct their refractive error. The sphere is found by neutralising the most *against* reflex, and the perpendicular meridian will then give a *with* reflex, which can be neutralised with plus cyls to give the sphero-cylindrical correction (which must be corrected for working distance).

Using negative cyls

This means that your retinoscopy result will be in a minus cyl format.

Identify the orientation of the two principal meridians, which will be perpendicular to each other. First, neutralise the most *with* reflex with plus spheres then neutralise the perpendicular *against* reflex with minus cyls. The lenses in the trial frame will give the retinoscopy result in minus cyl format, which must then be corrected for working distance.

Using spheres only

It is possible to obtain an objective refractive result without using any cylindrical lenses. Identify the two principal meridians. Neutralise one of the meridians with a sphere, record the result and orientation of reflex then remove the sphere. Following this, neutralise the perpen-dicular meridian with a sphere and record the result and orientation of the reflex. The refractive result can then be expressed in either plus or minus cyl format; in both cases, the magnitude of the cyl is the dif-ference between the two spheres. It can be useful to use a power cross to generate the resultant prescription.

Power crosses

As noted, if working in plus or minus cyls, the resultant refraction obtained by retinoscopy will simply be the lenses in the trial frame (this does not apply if working in spheres). This can then be corrected for working distance.

Therefore, it is not necessary to draw power crosses and power crosses are not required for the Refraction Certificate Examination (at the time of writing). However, since some practitioners use power crosses it is good practice to understand them. Furthermore, if you work only in spheres, it is useful to use a power cross to obtain your resultant refraction.

Each arrowed arm of a power cross represents the direction of movement of the retinoscope sweep. For example, when sweeping horizontally with the scope slit orientated vertically, the power in the horizontal plane (180) is examined. Therefore, if a sphere with power +3.50 dioptres neutralises a horizontal sweep, this implies the power in the horizontal direction is +3.50 dioptres. If a sphere with power +2.00 dioptres is then required to neutralise a vertical sweep with a horizontally orientated scope slit (to assess vertically acting power), the resultant power cross would be:

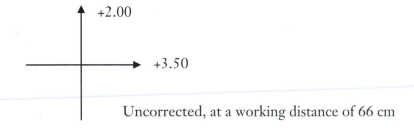

Uncorrected, at a working distance of 66 cm

Correcting for working distance would give:

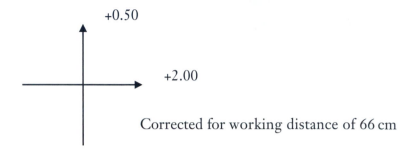

+0.50

+2.00

Corrected for working distance of 66 cm

To obtain the prescription from the power cross in positive cyl notation:
- record the least positive sweep as the sphere
- record the cyl as the difference between the two sweeps
- record the axis as the same axis of the most positive sweep (remembering that the axis is perpendicular to the direction of action of the power arrow).

Therefore, this example gives the prescription +0.50/+1.50 @ 090, which, when transposed, may also be written +2.00/−1.50 @ 180.

Here is another power cross example:

With slit at 045, power sweep at 135, a sphere of power −1.50 dioptres is required for neutralisation. With slit at 135, power sweep at 045, a sphere of power +0.25 dioptres is required for neutralisation. This gives the power cross:

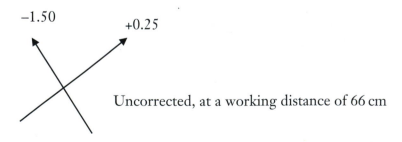

−1.50

+0.25

Uncorrected, at a working distance of 66 cm

Which, when corrected for working distance, gives:

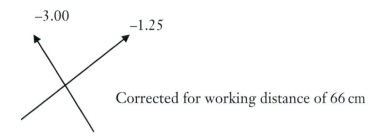

−3.00

−1.25

Corrected for working distance of 66 cm

Which gives the prescription −3.00/+1.75 @ 135.

Therefore, if working in plus or minus cyls, power crosses are not necessary since the resultant prescription, once corrected for working distance, is simply the lenses in the frame. However, if refracting in spheres, power crosses are useful for obtaining the prescription.

Interpreting the initial retinoscopy sweeps

When you are just starting, it is useful to have a clear idea in your mind of how to interpret the initial retinoscopy sweeps, since it is from here that you will make sequential decisions.

The level of your experience will become painfully obvious to the examiners at this early stage, so it is important to be confident and decisive at this point.

It is useful to make three sweeps: one with the slit vertical, one with it horizontal and one that is obliquely orientated at a meridian that has become clear to you following the vertical and horizontal sweeps, if there is an oblique reflex.

Assuming you are working at 66 cm and have decided to work in plus cyls format, consider the seven possible initial scope sweep results:

1   Neutralised in all meridians.
    The patient has a spherical refractive error of −1.50 dioptres (no cyl).
2   A dull, slow reflex that is difficult to interpret.
    Provided your retinoscope battery has not been exhausted from all

your enthusiastic work, the patient has a high degree of ametropia, so try interposing a ±5 or ±10 spherical lens. Remember, aphakia is a common cause of high hypermetropia.

3 An *against* reflex in all meridians that is equally fast and bright.
The patient is more myopic than –1.50 dioptres, and there is no significant astigmatism (neutralise with minus spheres).

4 A *with* reflex in all meridians that is equally fast and bright.
The patient is more plus than –1.50 dioptres, and there is no significant astigmatism (neutralise with plus spheres).

5 An *against* reflex in one meridian but more *against* (slower and duller) in another.
The patient has compound myopic astigmatism. Add minus spheres until the most *against* cyl is neutralised, leaving a perpendicular *with* reflex that can be neutralised with plus cyls.

6 A *with* reflex in one meridian but more *with* (slower and duller) in another.
The patient has compound hypermetropic (or rather more plus than –1.50 dioptres) astigmatism. Add plus spheres until the least *with* cyl (faster and brighter reflex) is neutralised leaving a perpendicular *with* reflex that can be neutralised with plus cyls.

7 A *with* reflex in one meridian and an *against* reflex in the perpendicular meridian.
The patient has mixed astigmatism. Add minus spheres to neutralise the *against* reflex then add plus cyls to neutralise the *with* reflex.

Cycloplegic versus non-cycloplegic retinoscopy

'Cycloplegia' refers to paralysis of the ciliary muscle, so that accommodation is not possible. Cycloplegics, such as topical cyclopentolate, will cause mydriasis (pupil dilatation) in addition to cycloplegia.

Non-cycloplegic retinoscopy is often sufficient for the majority of adult patients, especially if they are presbyopic (no effective accommodation). However, in the following situations it is useful to perform cycloplegic refraction:

● in children and young adults (especially if they are myopic) to remove accommodation, which gives a falsely myopic refraction if not removed

- in adults with small pupils or opaque media (such as a corneal scar or cataract) who have a poor-quality retinoscopic reflex without pupil dilatation.

Ensure that the cycloplegia is complete by instilling the cycloplegic and waiting at least 30 minutes. Check that there is no miosis following illumination of the pupil. Since cyclopentolate can sting, consider first giving a topical anaesthetic for children. Note that the pupil dilatation occurs before the full cycloplegic effect, so it is necessary to wait the full 30 minutes, even if the pupil is dilated after 10 minutes.

Other aspects of cycloplegic retinoscopy

- If the patient is a child (or an adult with learning disability), trial frames are not always tolerated. Try half-aperture child trial frames or simply place lenses in your own fingers in front of the child's eye.
- Children are less likely to remain still. The challenge here is to ensure your retinoscope light is on the visual axis of the child, since spurious astigmatism is noted if you are not co-axial to the eye. It is also harder to keep a constant working distance, which is typically shorter for a child (50 cm, with a –2.00 dioptre working distance correction) than for an adult (66 cm, with a –1.50 dioptre working distance correction).
- Neutralisation can be harder to appreciate. The direction of the initial retinoscopic reflex can be easier to determine in dilated eyes, but this can give a false sense of security, as the neutralisation point can be more difficult to establish. It may seem that neutralisation occurs over a wider range of lenses relative to non-cycloplegic refraction – it is important to watch the central reflex of the dilated pupil and 'push' the lenses until clear reversal is seen. For example, it may seem that neutralisation occurs at +2.00 dioptres, but do not settle for this – push the plus. It will

then become apparent, for example, that the central reflex gives a better neutralisation reflex at +3.00 dioptres and reversal is seen with +3.25 dioptres.

- Accommodation is not active – hence, there is no need for the patient to comply with distant fixation and there is no need to fog the fellow eye.

Other aspects of non-cycloplegic retinoscopy

- Trial frames are typically tolerated in adult non-cycloplegic retinoscopy, and these can help with establishing a more accurate angle of an astigmatic meridian.
- Patients are generally still. This makes it easier for your retinoscope's light to remain co-axial with the patient's eye, thus reducing the risk of spurious astigmatism.
- With small pupils or opaque media (such as a corneal scar or cataract), the reflex can be difficult to interpret. A dim room will dilate the pupil and help with this.
- Accommodation is active in pre-presbyopes (especially if myopic); this can be reduced by fogging the fellow eye adequately, maintaining distant fixation and avoiding prolonged retinoscopy bursts (try to make a decision within the first couple of sweeps and always within a few seconds).

Reducing accommodation in non-cycloplegic retinoscopy:
1 fog fellow eye
2 ensure patient maintains distant fixation
3 avoid prolonged retinoscopy bursts.

Failure to reduce accommodation gives a spuriously myopic result.

Finally, some important retinoscopy tips.

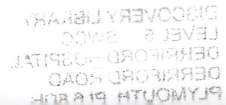

- Keep your lenses tidy (it will infuriate the examiners having to tidy up after you).
- Put your next lens into the trial frame before taking a lens out (this will help to minimise any accommodation).
- No retinoscopy sweep should last more than a few seconds. Prolonged sweeps not only induce accommodation (if non-cycloplegic) but also demonstrate to the examiners that you do not know how to act in response to what you see. Therefore, if you are not sure after a few seconds, come away, put a different lens in and try again.
- If the reflex is too dull to interpret, check your retinoscope battery. If the battery is OK, you are dealing with high ametropia. Try interposing a ±5 or ±10 sphere.
- If the results are too minus, check that the patient is not accommodating, either because they are not looking at the distant target (patients need constant reminders to do this) or because you have occluded rather than fogged the fellow eye. Occlude the fellow eye when checking visual acuity, but when using your retinoscope and for subjective refraction fog the fellow eye (with a +2 to +4 add on your estimated prescription to reduce accommodation). If the patient is amblyopic or diplopic, avoid fogging and simply occlude the fellow eye for retinoscopy and subjective refraction. If accommodation is an issue (as it is with all children), cycloplegic refraction is required.
- If the results are too plus, remember to subtract the working distance correction factor.

Subjective refraction

Subjective refraction involves the patient making conscious decisions so that a prescription that has been approximated by objective means (retinoscopy) can be fine-tuned.

Therefore, this is not always possible in children or patients with learning disability, so your retinoscopy result will provide the basis for spectacle prescription in these patients.

The process of subjective refraction should start within 10 minutes of the refractive process and take no longer than 10 minutes. The process includes the following stages:

1 refining the sphere
2 refining the cyl axis
3 refining the cyl power with sphere compensation
4 duochrome testing
5 binocular balance testing
6 MR and PCT
7 near vision testing.

The refinement of the sphere and cyl and duochrome test is completed first for the right eye then for the left eye.

Binocular balance is then tested with both eyes open.

The MR test (and possibly PCT) is used to assess the tendency of the eyes to dissociate, to establish if prisms are required to control a symptomatic tropia.

Following this, the near vision is corrected and tested with appropriate correction for the right then the left eye (test each eye independently).

Retinoscopy should be conducted in dim light. Subjective refraction should be conducted in good light – so, when you put your retinoscope down, turn the lights back on.

Ensure you have recorded your retinoscopy results (corrected for working distance) and the visual acuity that was obtained with these.

As with retinoscopy, during subjective refraction, it remains important to fog the fellow eye (or, if appropriate, occlude the fellow eye – *see* p. 37). This not only reduces accommodation in non-cycloplegic refraction but also ensures that the patient's answers to your subjective refraction questions are based entirely on the eye being examined.

In addition, as with retinoscopy, when changing a lens, always put the next lens into the trial frame before taking a lens out, to minimise accommodation.

Refining the sphere

Ask the patient to fixate on one of the letters on the lowest line of the acuity chart that they can see comfortably.

Ask the patient:

'Is that letter clearer with [place a +0.25 sphere in front of their eye] *or without the lens* [remove the +0.25 sphere] *or about the same?'*

If a response is not immediately given, after only a couple of seconds remove the lens, wait a couple of seconds, then re-offer them the lens and the question. Do not simply hold the lens up waiting for a decision, since the quality of the answer diminishes rapidly with time. If no response is succinctly given, it is likely that the letter remains about the same.

If the patient reports that the letter is better or about the same, add the plus lens to the frame and repeat.

If they report that the letter is worse with the plus lens, do not give the plus lens. Instead, now offer them a −0.25 sphere and ask them:

'Is that letter better, or just smaller and darker?'

This minus lens should only be offered for a brief moment to avoid accommodation. If they immediately report that the letter is better, add the −0.25 sphere to the trial frame and repeat. If they report that the letter is smaller and darker, check the acuity and move onto refining the cyl. If they report that the letter is worse (even though you did not ask them this), also check the acuity and move onto refining the cyl.

Noticing that a letter is smaller and darker rather than actually better can be difficult, and there is the danger of overcorrecting accommodating myopes. Therefore, be slightly reluctant to keep giving minus spheres to a myope (such experience comes with practise).

Note that when the −0.25 sphere is offered, only hold this up for a couple of seconds. If the patient does not make a decision quickly, remove the –0.25 sphere and re-offer them the lens and the question. Do not simply hold the lens up waiting for a decision, since the quality of the decision will decrease with time and, in the case of this minus lens, the patient will accommodate.

Using a ±0.25 sphere to refine the sphere is appropriate if the acuity is 6/9 or better. If the acuity is between 6/12 and 6/18, use a ±0.50 sphere, and consider using a ±1.00 sphere if it is worse than 6/18.

At this stage, do not panic if the acuity is poor and cannot be improved. It may be that the patient has a large cyl (a high degree of astigmatism). Therefore, move onto refining the cyl when an end point is reached, rather than persevering only with spheres in the pursuit of perfect acuity.

Refining the cyl axis

Refining the cyl follows refining the sphere.

The fogging of the fellow eye should remain in place and, for the purpose of the Refraction Certificate Examination, if demonstrating subjective refraction of the cylinder only, adequate fogging must first be ensured (*see* p. 37).

The cylindrical component of the spectacle prescription is fine-tuned subjectively using the Jackson cross cylinder (JCC), which was popularised by Edward Jackson (1893–1929).

The JCC is a sphero-cylindrical (toric) lens in which the power of the cylinder is twice the power of the sphere and of the opposite sign. The JCC is equivalent to superimposing two cylindrical lenses of equal power but opposite sign with their axes perpendicular to each other. The handle of the JCC is 45 degrees to the axes of the cyls. Since there are two perpendicular opposing cyls, an axis for the JCC is not denoted. The spherical equivalent (equal to the sphere plus half the cyl) of a JCC is therefore zero.

If a –0.25 cyl is superimposed perpendicularly with a +0.25 cyl the net result is equivalent to –0.25/+0.50 (when transposed equivalent to +0.25/–0.50). This would be a 0.50 JCC, since the JCC is defined by the power of the cyl notation.

JCCs are available in various powers, typically 0.50 and 1.00, and this is usually written on the shaft (*see* Figures 4.6 and 4.7). The power is named after the power of the cyl given by its notation. Hence a –0.25/+0.50 (same as +0.25 / –0.50) is a 0.50 JCC and a –0.50/+ 1.00 (same as +0.50 / –1.00) is a 1.00 JCC. The 0.50 JCC is used if acuity is 6/12 or better whereas the 1.00 JCC is used if acuity is worse than 6/12.

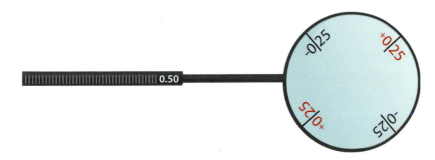

FIGURE 4.6 A 0.50 JCC (−0.25/+0.50)

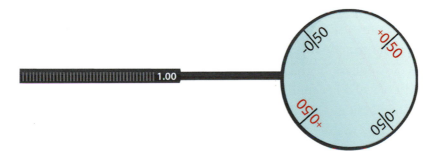

FIGURE 4.7 A 1.00 JCC (−0.50/+1.00)

Do not rely on the colour of the JCC axes to confirm which is plus and which is minus – the only way to be sure is to look at the lens markings. A 0.50 JCC will have +0.25 written on the lens and, perpendicular to this, –0.25 will be denoted. A 1.00 JCC will have +0.50 written on the lens and, perpendicular to this, –0.50 will be denoted. It should be acceptable to take your own JCCs to the examination if you wish.

To check the cyl axis (established by retinoscopy) with the JCC, hold the *handle along the proposed plus axis*. Ask the patient to look at the letter O (or other types of circular targets such as two double rings). Ask them:

> '*Does the O look rounder and clearer with lens 1* [position 1 – handle along axis] *or lens 2* [position 2 – twist 180 degrees] *or about the same?'*

Note that this question forces a comparison between the JCC in position 1 and the JCC position 2, *not* a comparison without the JCC. If the patient reports that both are equally as bad, this should be interpreted as meaning that position 1 is the same as position 2.

When working in plus cyls, if the patient prefers position 1, rotate the cyl so the axis moves towards the plus cyl of the JCC when in position 1.

If the patient prefers position 2, rotate the cyl so the axis moves towards the plus cyl of the JCC when in position 2.

The amount of rotation required (range 2 to 20 degrees in any alteration) depends upon the acuity and the strength of the cyl. If acuity is already good, only move the cyl by small amounts to avoid losing the good acuity. If the cyl is large, avoid large movements, since only a couple of degrees of movement of a large cyl can make quite a difference. This appreciation comes with practise. If unsure, apply the 'bracketing' technique, in which you initially move the axis by 20 degrees, then re-check and move by 10 degrees, then 5 degrees, then 2 degrees to reach the desired end point. Never underestimate how important it is to obtain the correct axis for a high-powered cyl.

If the patient reports that position 1 is the same as position 2 (or, as is quite common, appears to reject both of them) an *end point* has been reached and a satisfactory axis has been obtained. Now move onto refining the cyl power.

Refining the cyl power with sphere compensation

Ask the patient to focus again on the distant circular target.

When working in plus cyls, hold the *plus JCC axis over the plus cyl axis in the trial frame* (position 3 – this increases the cyl power).

Ask the patient to:

> 'Look at the O – does the O look rounder and clearer with lens 3 [position 3] or lens 4 [position 4 – twist 180 degrees, this places the minus JCC axis over the plus cyl axis in the trial frame to decrease the cyl power] or about the same?'

Again, the forced comparison is between the two positions of the cross cyl, and not a comparison with no cross cyl.

If position 3 is preferred, add +0.50 cyl to the plus cyl and add –0.25 sphere. This *sphere compensation* when adjusting the cyl ensures the spherical equivalent of the lenses is maintained (spherical equivalent = sphere + cyl/2). To maintain the spherical equivalent, the sphere must be changed by half the amount of the cyl and in opposite direction.

If position 4 is preferred, reduce the plus cyl power by 0.50 cyl and add +0.25 sphere to maintain the same spherical equivalent.

If the cyl power is changed (and sphere compensated), it is necessary to re-check the axis, then again challenge the cyl power. If you do not trust the cyl obtained, reduce the cyl (or remove if small) and see if the patient prefers this (i.e. test for rejection of cyl), since patients are more likely to prefer under rather than over astigmatic correction.

Continue this process until an *end point* is reached for both the cyl axis and cyl power (i.e. until the patient reports that position 1 is same as 2, and position 3 is same as 4).

Re-check the acuity then proceed to the duochrome test.

Duochrome test

This is a monocular subjective test to minimise accommodation whilst the distance prescription is worn, which is especially important in myopes.

If a myope is overcorrected (prescription too minus), they are effectively rendered hypermetropic and may experience asthenopia (eye strain) due to prolonged accommodation.

The principle of the duochrome test relies on chromatic aberration, which is where white light, when refracted at an optical interface, is dispersed into its different colours (wavelengths).

An emmetropic eye focuses distant yellow-green light (555 nm wavelength) perfectly onto the retina. Red and green light are used for the duochrome, since their wavelength foci straddle yellow-green light by equal amounts (about 0.4 dioptres on either side), with green being deviated more than red, since red has the longer wavelength (*see* Figure 4.8).

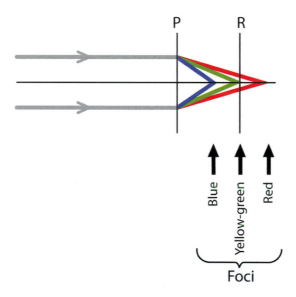

FIGURE 4.8 Dispersion and the human eye. Yellow-green light (555 nm) is focused perfectly onto the retina (R) by an emmetropic eye, when light is dispersed by the principal plane (P) of the optical interface. Green light falls in front of the retina and red light falls behind the retina by equal amounts

The duochrome consists of a ring of black circles or letters on a red and green background (*see* Figure 4.9).

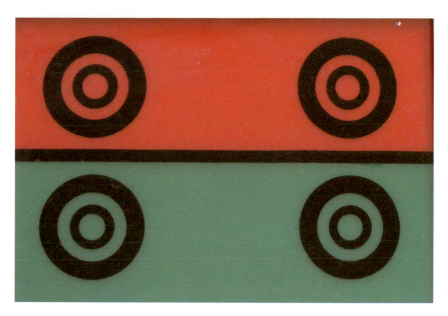

FIGURE 4.9 The duochrome

After the JCC test, whilst the fellow eye is still fogged, ask the patient to look at the distant duochrome and ask them if the circles/letters are clearer on the red, green or about the same. If they prefer green, add +0.25 sphere and repeat the question. Adding plus spheres should shift the preference from green to indifferent to red, and should relieve any accommodation with sacrificing the acuity.

Most practitioners would agree to leave myopes just on the red. For myopes, green is generally considered unacceptable, indifference (equal red and green) acceptable and just on the red preferable. The reason why myopes should not be left on the green is that they will be accommodating, as the prescription is too minus (i.e. overcorrected, rendering them hypermetropic).

This test is less important for hypermetropes – leave them indifferent or just on the green.

Note that the test can also be done in patients who are colour blind, since the test is dependent on the position of the image with respect to the retina. Therefore, colour-blind patients can be asked if the left or right (or upper or lower) rank is clearer, rather than the red or green rank.

Once adjusted, re-check the acuity.

As an extra step in myopes, it is useful to try the +1.00 blur back test, in which a +1.00 sphere is added that should blur the acuity to 6/12. If the myope remains 6/6, the prescription is too minus (overcorrected) and this +1.00 spherical lens should be added to their prescription to remove their accommodation, whilst retaining distance acuity.

The duochrome test is then repeated for the left eye (remember to fog the right eye).

Binocular balance

This is a final step to balance any accommodation and is done once both eyes have independently been subjectively refracted. It is particularly useful in young myopes to ensure that their prescription is too minus (overcorrected) and is an alternative to the +1.00 blur back test already described (see above).

Check the binocular acuity (remove any fogging or occluding lenses).

Now ask the patient to fixate on a letter on the lowest line that they can see.

Then place a +1.00 sphere over the left eye and a +0.25 sphere over the right eye and ask:

'Is the letter better, worse or about the same?'

If the letter is better or about the same, add the +0.25 sphere to the right eye and repeat. Do not give the plus lens if the letter appears worse (blurred).

Repeat the process with the +1.00 sphere over the right eye and the +0.25 sphere over the left eye.

If any lenses are added, re-check the binocular acuity to ensure that it has not reduced. If acuity has fallen, remove the plus lens.

Cover and alternate cover tests

These tests are useful in assessing the angle of deviation in eyes that have a squint or a tendency to drift.

It is important to understand these, since they are very quick to perform and often yield invaluable information. They also form a basic standpoint from which the PCT or MR test progresses from so that the squint can be quantified with prisms and prismatic incorporation can be considered in the spectacle prescription for significantly symptomatic patients.

Cover test

This is a quick test that is used to detect a manifest squint (tropia).

Remember that children (or adults with untreated childhood squint) with a manifest squint will suppress the image from the weaker, non-fixating eye and therefore not complain of diplopia. In contrast, adults with a recently acquired squint will complain of binocular diplopia that is worse when they look in the direction of extra-ocular muscle under-action.

The cover test should be performed:

- with and without spectacles
- with and without any compensatory head posture
- for distance and near (to torchlight and an accommodative target)
- always in the primary position and, if necessary, in the different directions of gaze.

For the distance cover test, ask the patient to fixate on a distant (6 m) target. Remember to first gently guide the patient's head into the primary position to remove any compensatory head posture.

Cover the left eye and observe for any movement in the right eye (*see* Figure 4.10).

- Esotropia (convergent squint) when the right eye initially is pointing nasally and then moves temporally on cover test.
- Exotropia (divergent squint) when the right eye initially is pointing temporally and then moves nasally on cover test.

- Right hyper-/hypo- tropia (vertical squint) when the right eye initially is higher/lower than the left and then moves downwards/upwards on cover test.

Right   Left

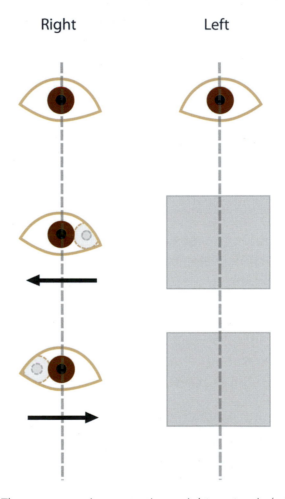

FIGURE 4.10 The cover test demonstrating a right esotropia (middle picture) and exotropia (bottom picture)

Now repeat the cover test with the right eye occluded, observing the movement of the left.

If there was movement with left eye occlusion but not for right eye occlusion, the tropia will be a 'right eye' tropia (e.g. right esotropia if the right eye moved temporally), since the left eye is the more stable eye that is adopting fixation (and vice versa for movement with right eye occlusion but not left eye occlusion).

Repeat the cover test with spectacles and with any compensatory head posture. Then repeat the cover test with a near torchlight followed by a near accommodative target, such as a small attention-holding image at 33 cm (reading distance).

Alternate cover test

The alternate cover test is a dissociative test that dissociates, or uncouples, the eyes. As each eye 'sees' a different fixation target, their true tendency to drift is released. As the alternate cover test continues, this tendency to drift often becomes more marked.

Therefore, the amount of deviation noted with the alternate cover test is the sum of the both the manifest squint (detected with the cover test) and the latent component of the squint (the tendency of the eyes to drift once dissociated). If the deviation is observed with the cover test alone, this is known as a '-tropia'. If there is no deviation with the cover test but there is with the alternate cover test, this isolated latent component is known as a '-phoria'.

As with the cover test, the alternate cover test should be performed:
- with and without spectacles
- with and without any compensatory head posture
- for distance and near (to torchlight and an accommodative target)
- always in the primary position and, if necessary, in the different directions of gaze.

For the distance alternate cover test, ask the patient to fixate on a distant (6 m) target. Remember to first gently guide the patient's head into the primary position to remove any compensatory head posture.

Cover the left eye and observe for any movement in the right eye. Then swiftly move the occluder to cover the right eye and observe for any movement as the left eye becomes uncovered. Repeat this a few times, until the degree of movement has settled (since it will increase with time) and once you have noted the direction of movement.

- A temporal movement (from initial nasal, convergent position) implies an esodeviation.
- A nasal movement (from an initial temporal, divergent position) implies an exodeviation.
- A down/up movement (from an initial high/low position) implies a hyper-/hypo- (vertical) deviation.

If the eyes rapidly take up fixation, this suggests the acuity and subsequent neural link with the visual pathways is similar for each eye. If one eye is slow to take up fixation (sometimes requiring verbal encouragement), it is likely that the acuity in this eye is poor.

Repeat the alternate cover test for near torchlight then a near accommodative target at 33 cm reading distance.

Prism cover test

The PCT allows the measurement of the angle of deviation, which allows objective quantification of the squint and subsequent prescription of the prism for symptomatic control if necessary.

As with the cover test, the PCT should be performed:

- with and without spectacles
- with and without any compensatory head posture
- for distance and near (the patient can hold the near accommodative target)
- always in the primary position and, if necessary, in the different directions of gaze.

Note that the PCT should be performed for distant and near accommodative targets and different prisms may be required for distance and near prescriptions, since patients tend to converge on near fixation. Since the examiner requires one hand to hold the prism bar and one hand to move the occluder, when testing the angle for a near accommodative target, it is necessary to ask the patient to hold, and look at, the accommodative target.

A prism can be held in front of either eye, since the angle of deviation relates to the angle *between* the eyes. If you are right-handed, you may find it easier to hold the occluder in your left hand and the prisms in your right hand. The prisms can be held individually or in the form of a prism bar – whichever you feel more comfortable with.

A combination of horizontal and vertical prisms may be needed. First, establish the horizontal angle. Once this is corrected, look specifically for a vertical deviation and superimpose vertical prisms on the horizontal prism to correct the vertical component.

Vertical deviations are typically smaller than horizontal deviations but, in the absence of suppression (such as with an acquired squint in an adult in the case of thyroid eye disease or cranial nerve 4 palsy), they are often more symptomatic due to the binocular fusion range being smaller vertically rather than horizontally.

Note that prisms will have a form of demarcation, such as a cross, at their base to help orientation.

For the distance PCT, ask the patient to fixate on a distant (6 m) target. Remember to first gently guide the patient's head into the primary position to remove any compensatory head posture.

Perform an alternate cover test as described (*see* p. 59).

Repeat the alternate cover test with a prism in place:
- for exodeviations, a base-in (BI) prism is needed
- for esodeviations, a base-out (BO) prism is needed
- for hyper-/hypodeviations, a base-down (BD)/base-up (BU) prism is needed.

There is no need to remember these listed points – just remember that the *correcting prism must have its apex pointing in the direction of deviation*.

If the movement is in the same direction with this corrective prism, the strength of the prism must be increased. If the movement has reversed direction, the prism strength must be reduced. The aim is to alter the prisms until reversal is noted, to obtain a satisfactory *end point*, which is when the eyes remain still during the alternate cover test since the prisms have neutralised any deviation. This can be confirmed by asking the patient if their double vision has been eliminated.

As mentioned, first correct the horizontal angle then look specifically for a vertical component and correct this, if present, by superimposing vertical prisms upon the correcting horizontal prism.

Now repeat the test for a near accommodative target (held by the patient at 33 cm reading distance). The patient should wear their near spectacles (albeit without prisms at this stage).

When incorporating prisms into the spectacle prescription, the term 'prism dioptre' can be denoted by a triangle (Δ). However, as this can be mistaken for a zero, it is safer to use the abbreviation 'pd' in the spectacle prescription. The amount of deviation in degrees is corrected by a prism with a power double that magnitude in prism dioptres. For example, a 15-degree angle of deviation is corrected by a 30 pd prism.

Typically, the prismatic correction is halved between the two lenses and the bases will be in the same direction for horizontal deviations and in opposite directions for vertical deviations. For example, a 13 pd exodeviation will be corrected by a 6 pd BI correction in front of the right eye and a 7 pd BI correction in front of the left eye. A 4 pd right hyperdeviation will be corrected by a 2 pd BD correction in front of the right eye and a 2 pd BU correction in front of the left eye.

> Remember that the apex of the correcting prism is always in the direction of squint deviation.

Maddox rod test

The Maddox rod (MR) test is a subjective assessment of extra-ocular muscle balance and estimates the degree of phoria (tendency of eyes to drift so they are not directed at the same target).

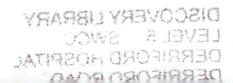

The majority of patients do not needs prisms. Prisms should only be incorporated into the spectacle prescription if:

- there is a history of double vision, or significant asthenopic (eye strain) symptoms, associated with a demonstrable phoria (latent squint)
- if a manifest squint (tropia) is noticed with the cover test
- restoration of orthophoria is achieved with the proposed prisms using the MR test (and PCT).

If there is no double vision and if no tropia is seen with a cover test, the MR test is unnecessary, as, regardless of what it shows, there will be no need for prismatic correction. Therefore, in the Refraction Certificate Examination, always consider that the correct answer might be to order no prisms.

You may find that some patients without any refractive correction have acuity that is too poor to allow them to appreciate multiple images. Without their spectacles, they do not complain of diplopia since everything is just simply blurred. In these cases, you will notice that once you have improved the acuity of both eyes the patient will start to complain of double vision. These patients will benefit from the MR test and prismatic control.

The MR consists of a series of strong, concave (plus) cylindrical red glass rods that convert the appearance of a white spot of light into a red streak (*see* Figure 4.11). When the rods are orientated vertically, the streak will be horizontal, and vice versa. Light from a distant source passes through the red cyls with no deviation in the same meridian as the axis of the cyls (since they have no power in the direction of their axis). Since there are multiple red rods, this gives a single red line on the retina and is perceived. Light rays in other meridians are converged by these powerful rods to a point focus just in front of the eye that is too close for it to be appreciated (this is not seen).

By placing the MR in front of one eye whilst the patient fixates at a distant white light, the two eyes are dissociated, since one eye stares at the red line whilst the other stares at the white light. If orthophoric,

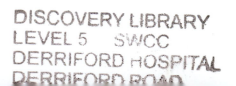

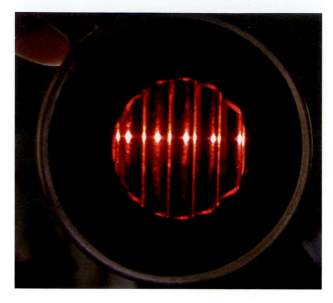

FIGURE 4.11 The Maddox rod consists of red cylinders. Here the Maddox rod is held with the rods orientated vertically, and this results in a horizontal red line of light, when light from a distant source is viewed through the Maddox rod

the red line will appear to pass through the white light when the red line is orientated either vertically or horizontally. If there is a horizontal phoria, when the red line is orientated vertically (rods horizontal), the red line will appear to one side. If there is a vertical phoria when the red line is orientated horizontally (rods vertical), the red line will appear either above or below the white light.

This may sound complex, but, with practise, the MR test can be completed in less than 1 minute with ease. Remember that corrective prisms have their apexes directed in the direction of eye deviation.

The distant cover test is useful to do prior to the MR test, since it gives an objective starting point that the MR test subjective result should match.

Now turn the room lights down. Ensure the patient is wearing their binocular, distance prescription and ask them to fixate at a distant white dot light (somebody holding a pen torch at the end of the room is sufficient if no white dot light is in the light box).

Hold the MR in front of the right eye with the bars orientated horizontally and ask the patient if they can see a vertical red line. If they cannot, occlude their left eye momentarily and they will usually see the red line. Ask them if the red line is to the right, left or straight through the white dot.

If the line goes through the white dot, no prismatic correction in the horizontal plane is required.

If the line is to the right, they have an esophoria, so BO prisms should be placed in front of the left eye until the red line is through the white spot. In theory, a BO prism could also be placed in front of the right eye to correct an esophoria, but because the MR is in front of the right eye, it is easier to place prisms in front of the left eye.

If the line is to the left, they have an exophoria, so BI prisms should be placed in front of the left eye until the red line is through the white spot. Again, this could also be corrected with a BI prism in front of the right eye, but as the MR is in front of the right eye, it is easier to place prisms in front of the left eye.

A 3 pd lens can be used first to try to shift the position of the red line to pass through the white spot or, if overcorrected, to pass over to the other side. In patients without diplopia, 3 pd is usually sufficient to shift the line and confirms that no prisms need to be incorporated into the spectacle prescription. In patients with diplopia, more than 3 pd will probably be required to shift the red line to pass through the white spot. The resultant prismatic correction should then be shared between the two eyes. For example, if 8 pd BO is required to correct an esodeviation, 4 pd BO in front of the right eye and 4 pd BO in front of the left eye should be prescribed. If 13 pd BI is required to correct an exodeviation, 7 pd BI in front of the right eye and 6 pd BI in front of the left eye should be prescribed.

Now hold the MR in front of the right eye with the rods orientated vertically and ask the patient if they can see a horizontal red line. Ask them if the red line is above, below or straight through the white light.

If the line goes through the white dot, no prismatic correction in the vertical plane is required.

If the line lies above the white dot, they have a left hyperdeviation, which can be corrected with a BD prism in front of the left eye. This could also be corrected with a BU prism in front of the right eye.

If the line lies below the white dot, they have a left hypodeviation, which can be corrected with a BU prism in front of the left eye (or a BD prism in front of the right eye).

Again, for vertical deviations, a 3 pd lens can be used, but note that patients are generally more sensitive to vertical deviations. For example, a 3 pd deviation in the horizontal plane is usually fused and does not result in symptomatic diplopia, whereas 3 pd in the vertical plane may not be fused and the patient may have diplopia. If a vertical prismatic correction is required, again this should be shared between the two eyes; however, unlike for horizontal deviations, in vertical deviations the prisms are orientated in opposite directions. For example, a 5 pd left hyperdeviation can be managed with 3 pd BD in front of the left eye and 2 pd BU in front of the right eye.

You may have realised that if the MR is placed in front of the right eye and the corrective prisms are then placed in front of the left eye, the apex of the prism is always in the same direction that the patient reports the red line to appear, relative to the white dot:

- line to the left: place prism with apex to left
- line to the right: place prism with apex to right
- line above: place prism with apex upwards
- line below: place prism with apex downwards.

Therefore, it is simple to place the MR in front of the right eye and use corrective prisms in front of the left eye with the apex pointing to where the red line lies. The only situation in which this is not possible is when the right eye has relatively poor best corrected acuity (due to amblyopia or ocular pathology). In this case, the MR should be held in front of the left eye.

Near vision

'Accommodation' refers to the process of the focal point of the eye shifting from a distant target to a near target.

Patients who are presbyopic are unable to read clearly whilst wearing their distant spectacle prescription due to an inability to accommodate.

Presbyopia manifests at an earlier age in hypermetropes (from age 35 years) than in emmetropes (from age 40 years) and may not ever manifest in myopes.

Near vision is also improved by pupillary constriction, which increases the depth of focus. Adequate macular function is also vital for satisfactory near vision. For these reasons, checking near vision with good illumination is most helpful.

Given that patients will converge with near targets, they may also require a prismatic correction different to their distant correction (*see* 'Prism cover test', p. 60).

To estimate an initial near add, obtain a brief relevant history:

- their age
- whether they have had previous cataract surgery with an intra-ocular lens implant (pseudophakia)
- their activities of daily living that involve near visual tasks – reading, needle work, model making, etc., since this will alter their near working distance.

The following guide should be a useful starting point.

Age	Near add
40–50 years	+1.00 to +1.50
50–60 years	+1.50 to +2.00
>60 years	+2.00 to +3.00
Pseudophakia	+2.50 to +3.00

To assess near vision, ask the patient to hold the reading chart at the comfortable near working distance for the near task they would like correction for; for example:

- reading – typically, about 33 cm

- needle work, model making, etc. – may be much closer and, therefore, require a greater near add
- computer work – such an intermediate distance may require a weaker add to the distant prescription, relative to full near correction required for reading.

Occlude the left eye and ask them to read the smallest print they can on the N-series reading chart held at their working distance. Now add the appropriate near plus lens and record the corrected near acuity (aiming for N5 or N6 in the absence of ocular disease).

Ask the patient to look at a letter then ask:

> '*Is the letter clearer with* [place a +0.25 sphere in front of their eye] *or without the lens* [remove the +0.25 sphere] *or about the same?*'

If they report that the letter is better with the lens or about the same, add the +0.25 sphere and repeat until acuity is optimal.

Repeat the process for the left eye (occlude the right) then check that the reading speed is good with both eyes not occluded.

The patient's near add is typically the same for both eyes, but this should still be checked because pre-presbyopes that have had unilateral cataract surgery will require a high near add in their pseudophakic eye and perhaps only a small near add in their phakic eye.

5

Retinoscopy of a model eye

The Refraction Certificate Examination may require you to complete objective refraction (retinoscopy) of a model eye within 5 minutes.

The model eye is on a simple stand and, fortunately, has been made to provide a scope reflex that is easier to interpret than real reflexes. However, since no trial frame can be used here, you need to take care when judging the working distance and in being aware of the cylindrical axis. This situation is similar to performing retinoscopy on children (who are averse to trial frames).

See Chapter 4 to learn how to use the retinoscope.

If working in plus cyls, refract the model eye using spheres until the least *with* movement is neutralised and leave a residual *with* movement in the perpendicular axis. Then place a plus cyl lens in front of the sphere (holding both lenses flush together) and rotate the cyl axis line so that it is orientated parallel to your scope slit. Continue to refract in this meridian until neutralised.

Great care must now be taken when recording your results. An approximation of the cyl axis must be made, since there is no trial frame to aid your recording of the cyl axis.

Furthermore, even if your working distance is typically 66 cm for refracting adults in trial frames, you will probably find that your working distance for refracting children without trial frames (and, therefore, model eyes) is reduced to 50 cm. If your working distance is 50 cm, it is necessary to add –2.00 sphere to your prescription to correct for working distance (rather than the –1.50 sphere that is added for a working distance of 66 cm).

Remember to state your working distance and its correction for the examiners. For example, if the retinoscopy gives –3.50/+1.75 @ 130, record your result as –5.50/+1.75 @ 130, corrected for a working distance of 50 cm.

6

How to use a focimeter

Focimeter principles

The focimeter is used to measure the back vertex power of a lens. It is possible to establish the sphere, cyl (power and axis) and near add of a pair of bifocal spectacles. It can also be used to measure any prisms that may have been incorporated into the lens. It is not so accurate at measuring the strength of varifocal spectacles.

The Refraction Certificate Examination requires you to use the focimeter. In 5 minutes, you will be expected to record the distance and near prescription for a pair of bifocal spectacles.

Focimeters have a diverging light source that passes through a card that has a ring of holes in and then to a collimating lens that converges light, which, once focused, gives a ring of dots. This ring of dots is observed through a viewing system. When the lens to be tested is placed on the focimeter, the distance of the card from the collimating lens can be altered until the dots are focused, and this gives a power value that is noted from a calibrated scale.

Although there are different types of focimeter, essentially, they all work according to this principle. If possible, try to become acquainted with at least two different types of focimeter (*see* Figure 6.1). In the examination, there is usually a couple of the commonly used focimeters to choose from.

Before using the focimeter, look at the spectacles and note that if they are bifocal a near add value will also be required. Quickly note that if they minify an object, they will be the spectacles of a myope (minus lens), whereas if they magnify an object then they will be the spectacles of hypermetrope (plus lens).

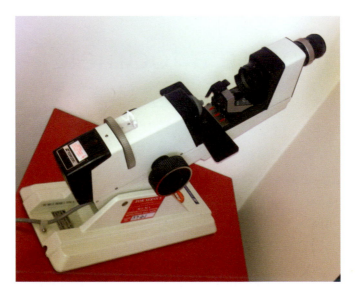

FIGURE 6.1 A focimeter

Recording distance prescription

Turn the focimeter on and set the focusing wheel to zero. Then turn the viewing eyepiece fully anticlockwise and look down the eyepiece, turning it clockwise until the dots and graticule are in focus (this reduces instrument accommodation, which will give a false recording).

Place the spectacles on the focimeter with the arms facing backwards, to ensure that the focimeter measures the back vertex power of the lens. Conventionally, the distance then near prescriptions are established for the right lens and then for the left lens.

If the spectacles are bifocals, check that it is the upper distance segment that is orientated on the focimeter. You may need to move the lens around until the ring of dots is centralised on the graticule. If this is not possible, this is due to a prism in the lens (*see* p. 75).

Once the spectacles are placed on the focimeter, a ring of dots is only seen if the lens only contains a sphere and when the collimating lens is focused. Therefore, rotate the focusing wheel until a crisp ring of dots is seen then note the power value and sign (+ or –) on the wheel. This will give the distance spherical prescription.

As with most cases, the prescription will have an astigmatic element, so, rather than a ring of dots being observed, a ring of fine lines is observed. Turning the focusing wheel will bring these lines into focus and turning the wheel further will bring a set of perpendicular lines into focus (the previous lines will become blurred or will disappear). It is necessary to adjust the axis of the graticule so that the lines are made linear. Once the axis has been corrected, turn the focusing wheel to bring the lines into sharp focus. Failure to first match the axis will result in an inability to sharply focus the lines. Record the power and the axis – this is the value of the cylindrical component in one of the two principal meridians. Then turn the focusing wheel until the perpendicular lines appear. Again, fine-tune the axis of the graticule until the lines are linear then alter the focus wheel until in sharp focus. Record the power and axis of this perpendicular principal meridian.

It is quite simple to convert the two cyl recordings into a spectacle prescription. If working in plus cyls:
- the sphere is the most negative recording
- the cyl is plus and is the *difference* between the two recordings
- the axis is the same as the most plus recording.

Some examples follow.

Two cyl recordings from focimeter	Prescription
+3.00 @ 030, –2.00 @ 120	–2.00/+5.00 @ 030
–1.75 @ 145, –3.25 @ 055	–3.25/+1.50 @ 145
+1.50 @ 060, +6.25 @ 150	+1.50/+4.75 @ 150

Note that the focimeter records the cyl axis and not the orientation of the cyl power (perpendicular to the axis). This is important to appreciate if using power crosses to obtain the prescription, rather than the simple three-step process described here.

For example, if the two cyl recordings from the focimeter are +3.00 @ 135 and –1.75 @ 045, this would give the following power cross:

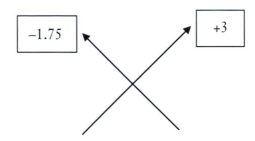

This gives –1.75/+4.75 @ 135 (equivalent to +3.00/–4.75 @ 045).

See 'Power crosses', in Chapter 4, to see how to obtain the prescription from the power cross. Although academically it is useful to appreciate power crosses, you may well find it practically simpler to use the three-step method already detailed.

Recording near add value

To measure the near add of the bifocal segment, move the spectacles so that the lower near segment is orientated on the focimeter. Rotate the focus wheel until the dots (or lines in the case of astigmatism) are in focus and record the power. Subtract the distance prescription from this near value to give the near add.

For example, if the dots are in sharp focus at –3.00 sphere for the distance segment and –1.50 sphere for the near segment, the near add will be +1.50 sphere. When establishing the near add for a sphero-cylindrical lens (used to correct astigmatism) ensure that the lines brought into focus are at the same orientation as those lines used to give the power value for distance that is subtracted from the near recording. For example, if the lines are in focus for the distance segment at +3.00 @ 030 and −2.50 @ 120 and the 030 line is in focus at +5.00 for the near segment, the near add is +2.00 sphere. The 120 lines would then be in focus at −0.50 for the near segment.

In most cases, the near add value will be the same for each eye. However, do not assume this, since they may be the spectacles of a young (pre-presbyopic) patient that has had unilateral cataract surgery. In this case, a near add may not be required on the eye that has not had surgery; however, a near add may be required on the side that has had cataract surgery.

Recording the prismatic correction

When trying to centre the dots on the graticule, it may become apparent that the dots cannot be centralised. This is due to a prism being incorporated into the lens.

The dots will be deviated towards the base of the prism because, although prisms deviate images towards their apex, the focimeter eyepiece viewing system inverts this view. The power of the prism is equal to the number of spaces (denoted by the graticule) that the dots are deviated.

For example, if the dots are deviated by two spaces upwards, there is a 2 pd BU prism in that lens. If the dots are deviated by four spaces to the right when the right lens is being assessed, there is a 4 pd BI prism in that lens.

Typically, the prismatic correction is halved between the two lenses, and the bases will be in the same direction for horizontal deviations and opposite directions for vertical deviations. For example, a 13 pd exodeviation will be corrected by a 6 pd BI correction in front of the right eye and 7 pd BI correction in front of the left eye. A 4 pd right hyperdeviation will be corrected by a 2 pd BD correction in front of the right eye and a 2 pd BU correction in front of the left eye. The apex of the correcting prism is always in the direction of deviation.

Symptomatic ocular deviations can be corrected by incorporating prisms into the spectacle prescription, which can be measured by the focimeter as described earlier. However, it is important to note that ocular deviations can also be controlled in another way – through 'lens decentration'. This is where the optical axis of the lens is purposefully decentred relative to the patient's pupil. The prismatic power (pd) is equal to the power of the lens (dioptres) multiplied by the distance of decentration (cm). If this has been done, it will still be possible to centre the image on the focimeter. Such prismatic correction could, therefore, be overlooked. The only way to detect lens decentration is by checking the lens for a marking that indicates this or by using a lens marker to mark the position of the pupil centre whilst the patient is wearing the spectacles. This mark should then be placed in the centre of the focimeter stop and any decentration will be evident. Fortunately, in the Refraction Certificate Examination, since you are only provided with a pair of bifocal spectacles and not with their owner, you are not expected to mark the pupil centre and assess for lens decentration.

7

Lens neutralisation

It is possible to establish the spectacle distance and near prescription (and also prismatic component) of a pair of bifocal spectacles using a lens box according to the principle of lens neutralisation. This estimate may not be as accurate as that established using a focimeter, but lens neutralisation is still a useful skill to have and one that is assessed in the Refraction Certificate Examination.

'Lens neutralisation' means using lenses that are equal in magnitude but opposite in direction to neutralise the spectacles, so there is no overall effect. For example, a +2.50 sphere in a spectacle lens is neutralised with a −2.50 spherical trial frame lens. A 2 pd BO prism will be neutralised by a 2 pd BI prism.

First, to establish if the lens is minus or plus, complete the transverse test. Pass the lens horizontally from right to left across a vertical line. If the image of the line moves in the same direction (right to left) as the sweep ('with'), the lens is minus. If the image of the line moves in the opposite direction to the sweep ('against'), the lens is plus. You may also notice that minus lenses will minify objects and plus lenses will magnify.

If the transverse test implies the test lens is minus, place a plus lens (say, +3.00 sphere) in direct contact and see if this eliminates the movement of the vertical line image. If the movement is still *with* the sweep, try a more plus lens; if it is *against*, try a less plus lens. The reverse is true for plus test lenses. Neutralisation occurs when the image of the vertical line remains still as the lenses are swept across them horizontally.

Note that it is vital that lenses are held in close contact, since if they are held apart their effective power is altered.

Once the lens has been neutralised, the prismatic component (if present) can be neutralised in the same fashion by the application of equal and opposite prisms. Images viewed through a prism are displaced towards their apex. Hence, a 3 pd BU prism will shift the image downwards and be neutralised by a 3 pd BD prism. Neutralisation occurs when the image is not shifted at all by the combined prisms.

8

Final tips for the exam

More than 2 months before the exam

Read this book!

Read the Refraction Certificate Examination application details very carefully and contact the Royal College if you have any uncertainties about what is expected of you.

Consider attending a course on refraction. This will no doubt be helpful, but they are expensive and absolutely no substitute for refracting yourself.

Get study leave – not just for the exam but for the week before the exam, during which time you must refract intensively.

Get refracting! Print out Appendix 1, 'Typical refractive recording sheet', and fill in for each person you refract. Keep all these sheets so you can keep a record of how many you have done and what you have learnt from each one.

Ideally, get your own retinoscope and borrow a decent trial frame and JCCs so that you are familiar with the equipment that you will use in the examination.

One month before the exam

By now, you will probably have realised that the main limitation to practising is obtaining a free room and a subject to refract. It does not take long to refract everybody in the department, so you will need to look elsewhere.

Try all staff – this includes medical, nursing, health care assistants, students and administrative staff. Another option is to refract patients whilst they are waiting to be seen during clinic.

Aim to refract patients of all ages (children, pre-presbyopic adults, presbyopic adults) and with different characteristics (high myopia, high hypermetropia or aphakia, those with significant astigmatism, those that need prismatic control, small pupils, clear phakic lenses, those with cataract and pseudophakic patients).

Remember to practice both non-cycloplegic and cycloplegic refraction.

Finally, consider booking people in advance into 30-minute slots to refract during your study week to ensure a final burst of resources!

One week before the exam

Concentrate on getting your numbers up by refracting the people that you have booked into your free study week.

Re-confirm that you understand the examination format.

Check you have all the things you will need for the examination:

- your own retinoscope (place fresh batteries in this and take a spare pair)
- a borrowed trial frame and JCCs
- an occluder, rule and pen torch (for the cover test)
- your passport or driving licence (required by examiners to confirm your identity)
- all the examination, accommodation and travel details

On the day

Prepare for starting with any station first.

Remember to be consistent when recording your results – always use only positive cyls or only negative cyls (do not use both positive and negative cyl nomenclature). Always specify the working distance and correct for this.

All dioptric powers should be to two decimal places and have a clear + or − sign (e.g. +0.25, −1.50). The degree symbol (°) should be avoided and all axes should be to three significant figures (e.g. 045, 010, 135).

Keep your lenses tidy – it will annoy the examiners if they have to tidy up after you.

If you find yourself struggling with a retinoscopy reflex, do not just sit there persisting, as prolonged retinoscopy sweeping is uncomfortable for the patient, induces accommodation and demonstrates to the examiners your uncertainty. No retinoscopy sweep burst should take longer than a few seconds, so try to make a decision and simply come away and try a different lens if you are unsure.

Before formally starting, check that you are comfortable with the room set-up (lighting, record sheet and equipment) then ask questions if you are uncertain before the bell actually goes.

Good luck!

Jonathan C Park and David H Jones

Typical refractive recording sheet

Name: ....

Age: ....

Occupation/Hobbies/Ophthalmic history: ....

	RIGHT	**LEFT**
Unaided visual acuity (VA)		
Pinhole VA		
Unaided near VA		
IPD distance		
IPD near		
BVD		
RETINOSCOPY		
Working distance		
SUBJECTIVE REFRACTION		
PRESCRIPTION		

RIGHT	Sph	Cyl	Axis	Prism	Base		Sph	Cyl	Axis	Prism	Base	LEFT
						Dist.						
						Near						

CORRECTED VA ....

DISTANCE ....

NEAR ....

The retinoscope

There are two types of retinoscope – slit and spot. Slit retinoscopes are far more common in ophthalmic outpatient departments, so the principles of the slit retinoscope are detailed here.

A retinoscope consists of a light source and a mirror with a viewing hole in it so the observer can observe whatever is illuminated when looking through the hole.

When the cuff of the slit retinoscope is fully down, a linear light is produced (the scope slit). With the cuff down (correct position), a condensing lens between the light and mirror allows diverging rays to exit the retinoscope (*see* Figure A2.1). With the cuff upwards, the condensing lens is moved to a different position to give converging rays.

As the scope slit is swept across the pupil, light entering the patient's eye is reflected by the retina then refracted by their eye before being observed by the practitioner through the viewing hole of the retinoscope. The quality of the light reflex depends upon the following factors:

- cuff position
- working distance
- refractive state of the patient's eye
- orientation of retinoscope slit and direction of sweep.

By ensuring that the cuff is fully down, the working distance is known and the scope slit orientation and direction of sweep are controlled, it is possible for the practitioner to obtain an objective refraction for the patient's eye by interspersing various trial lenses to neutralise the retinoscopy reflex (*see* Chapter 4).

The optics of the retinoscope can be detailed further by considering how the retina is illuminated (illumination stage), how an image of the illuminated retina is formed at the patient's far point (reflex stage) and how the image at the far point is located by moving the illumination across the retina and noting the reflex quality (projection stage).

We recommend that for further detailed optics information you refer to this excellent book, which is also very useful for the Royal College of Ophthalmologists' Part 1 Fellowship Examination:

Elkington AR, Frank HJ, Greaney MJ. *Clinical Optics*. 3rd ed. London, Malden, MA, and Victoria: Blackwell; 2006.

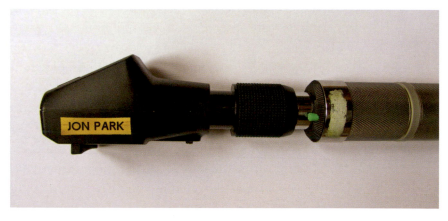

FIGURE A2.1 A retinoscope with the cuff down

Index

Entries in **bold** denote figures and tables.